Moods in Motion

A Coloring and Healing Book for Postpartum Moms

by

Karen Kleiman, MSW, LCSW

Illustrations by Lisa Powell Braun

INTRODUCTION

It's hard being a mother.

Even the good days are sprinkled with worry and unpredictability. On bad days, it can feel utterly overwhelming.

As a therapist who has specialized in the treatment of prenatal and postpartum anxiety and depression for over thirty years, I've had the privilege of sharing the journey with hundreds of women as they transition into the world of motherhood. There is often tremendous joy, and there is also great suffering.

Recently, I became intrigued by the trending popularity of adult coloring books. There is increasing evidence that health benefits associated with coloring activities are actually similar to meditation. This is because coloring can help block out negative thoughts by giving the brain something else to focus on. Unfortunately, negative, unwanted thoughts are common in motherhood. Even though these thoughts can be incredibly unsettling, they are associated with anxiety which means they can be decreased by distracting your brain. In this way, coloring is a restorative tool for distress!

HOW TO USE THIS BOOK

I tried hard to reconcile the light-hearted nature of this book with the seriousness of postpartum depression and anxiety. I am hopeful that together with Lisa's illustrations, we have achieved a balance of combining a playful and purposeful activity, with the seriousness of your experience.

The unique structure of this book addresses specific symptoms of postpartum depression and anxiety. The **Symptom Page** illustrates how a symptom might be perceived by a woman, directly followed by a **Healing Page**. Each Healing Page provides an affirmation or recommendation which has been shown to benefit postpartum women in distress. In this way, *Moods in Motion* is more than a coloring book which will distract your brain and ease your stress. It is an illustrated guide toward healing which provides an opportunity for you to actively participate in your recovery.

I wish you each a smooth transition. Remember to let someone know how you are feeling and ask for help if you need it.

Try to include some coloring time in your occasional moments of peace and quiet...it will help you feel better.

Warmly,

ABOUT KAREN KLEIMAN
Karen Kleiman, MSW, LCSW, is a well-known international expert on the treatment of postpartum depression and anxiety. She is the author of "This Isn't What I Expected" and several other books on postpartum distress and recovery.
postpartumstress.com

"What happened to the old me? I just don't feel like myself."

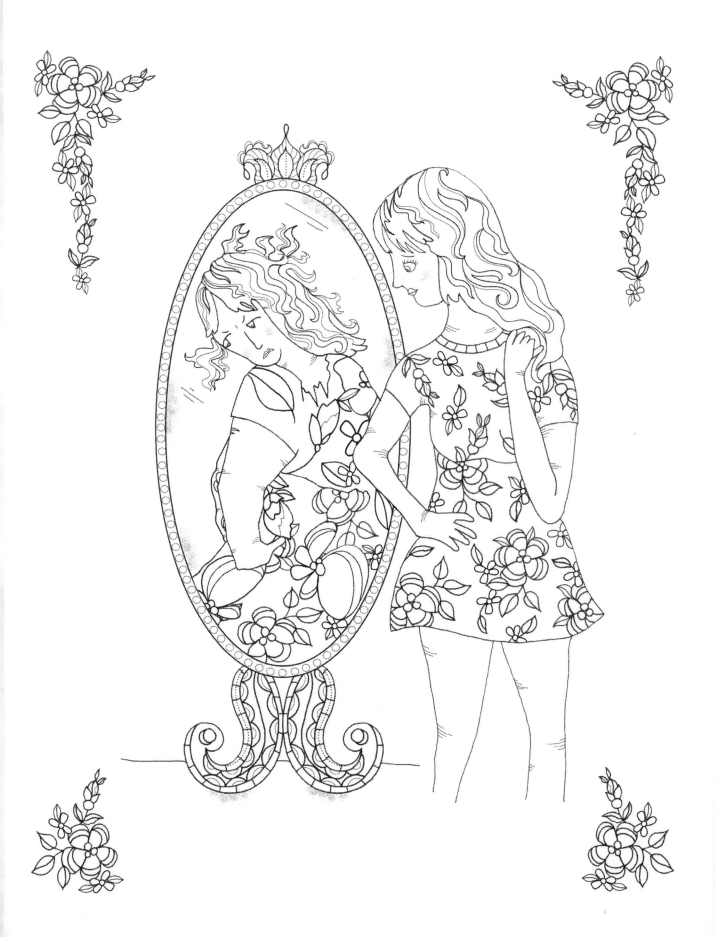

You are still you. Your symptoms are in the way right now.
It feels like this is who you are, but it's not.
These are symptoms.
You can do what you need to do, and be yourself,
even if you have symptoms.

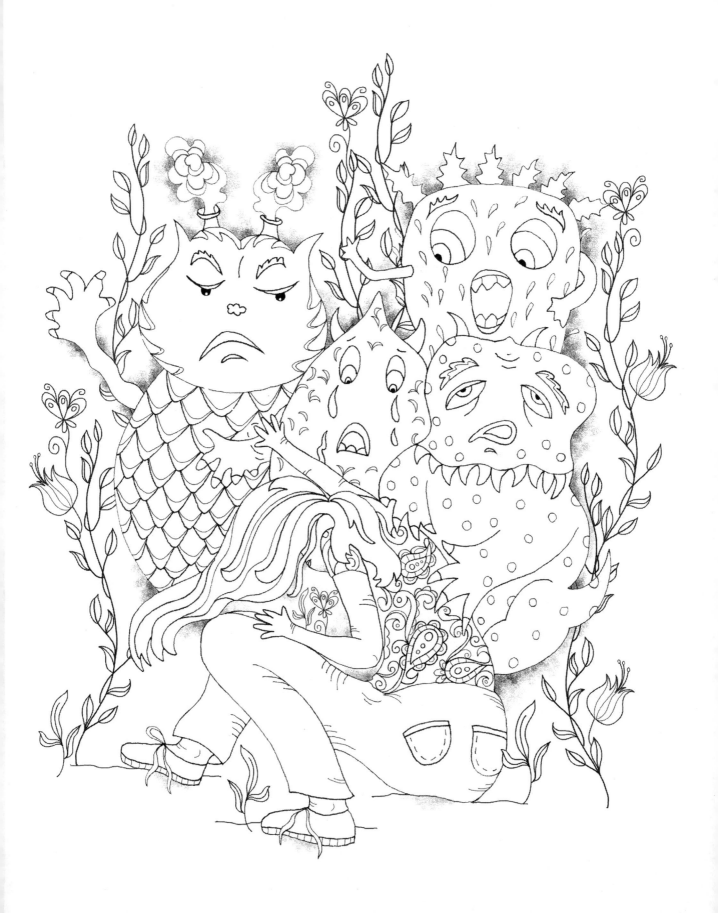

"I feel sad and tearful all the time."

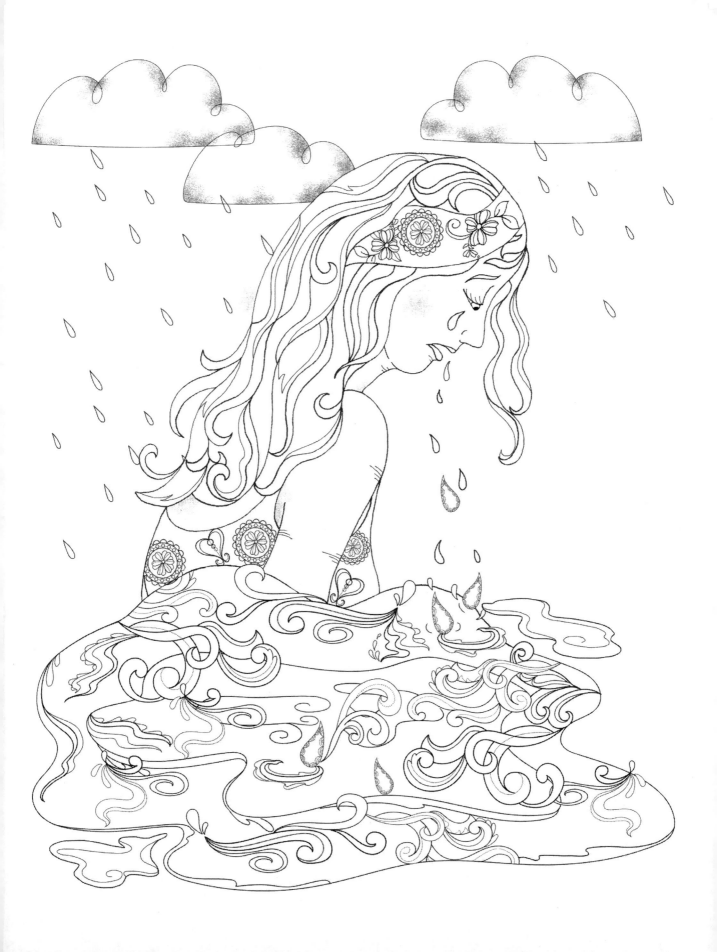

Cry. It's okay.
You cannot control everything.
Accept your symptoms with self-compassion.
Be kind to yourself.

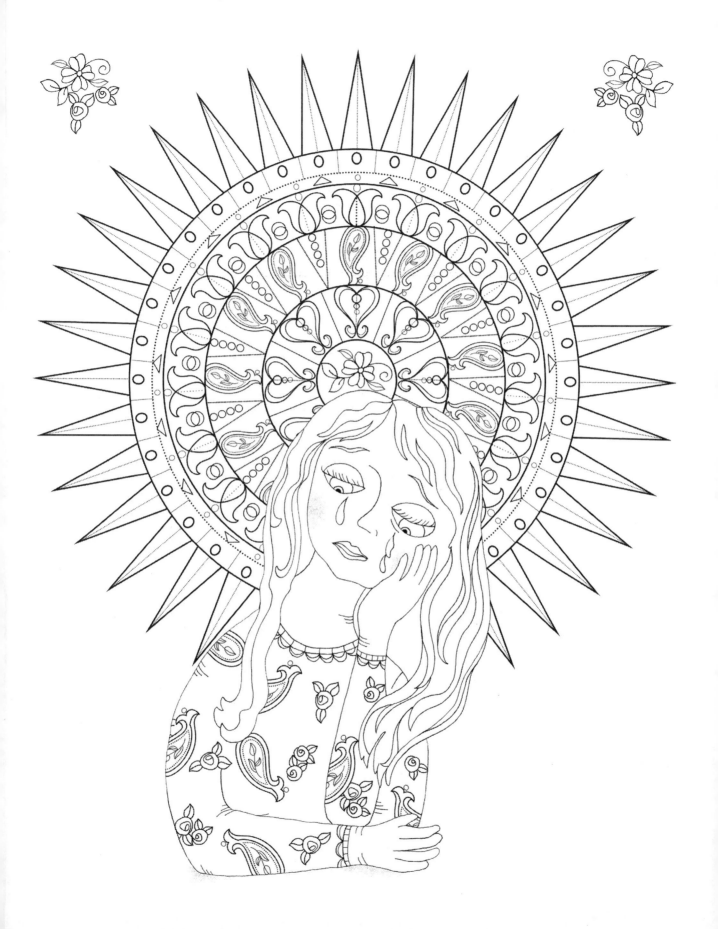

"I am having scary thoughts that I'm afraid to tell anyone."

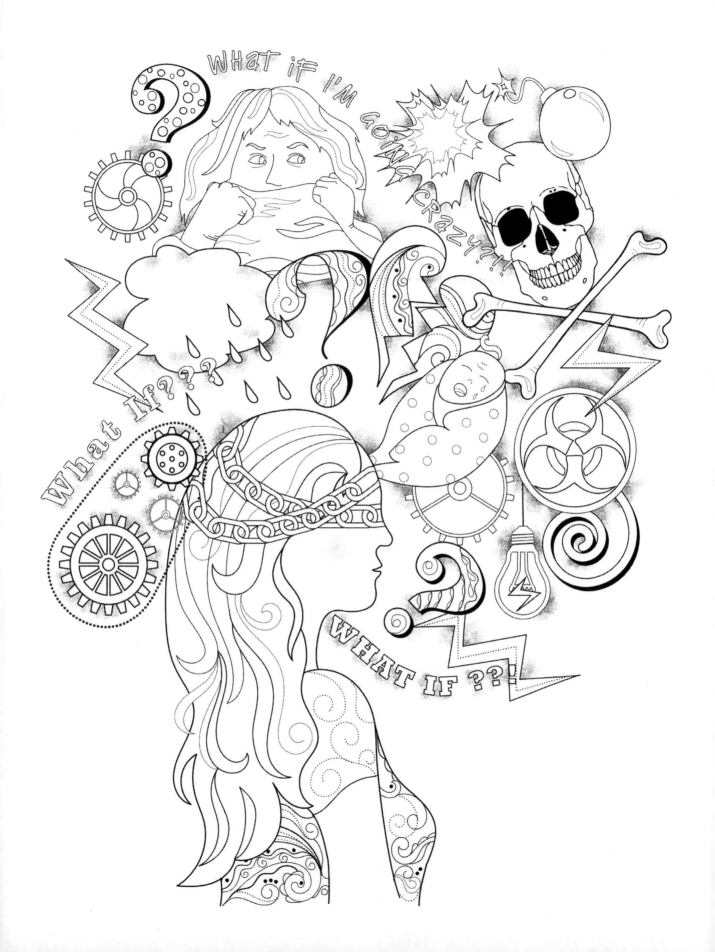

If your thoughts are scaring you, they are signs of anxiety.
Everything is okay.
Anxious thoughts get scarier when you try to push them away.
Talk to someone you trust.
Tell your provider. Tell your partner.
Write the thoughts down.
Once you acknowledge that they are there, they will lose power.
Notice them. Let them go.

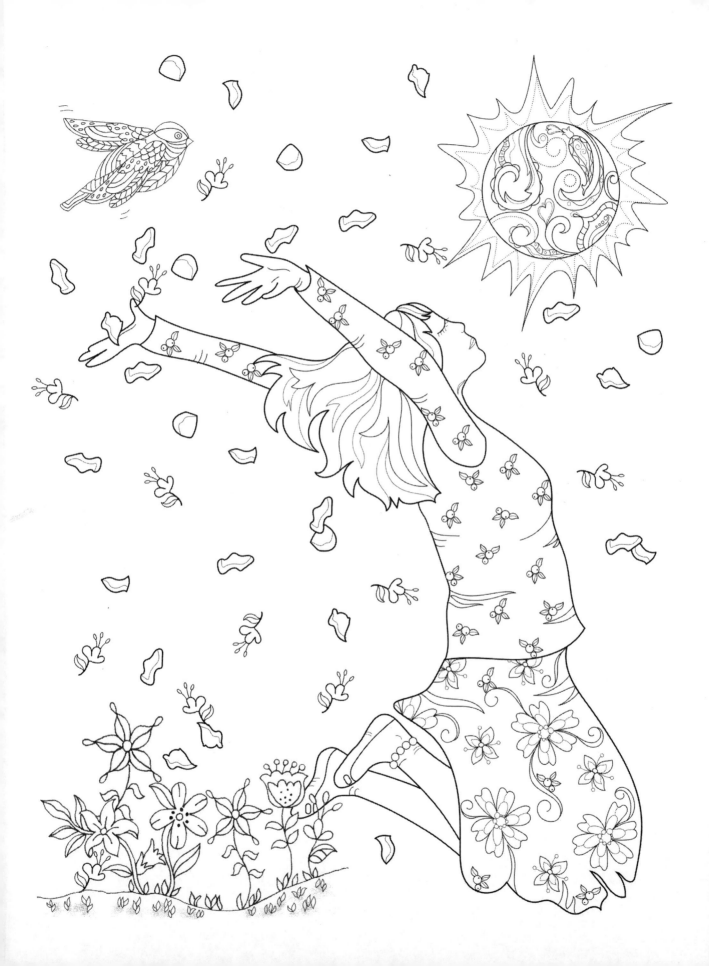

"I have no appetite. I cannot sleep."

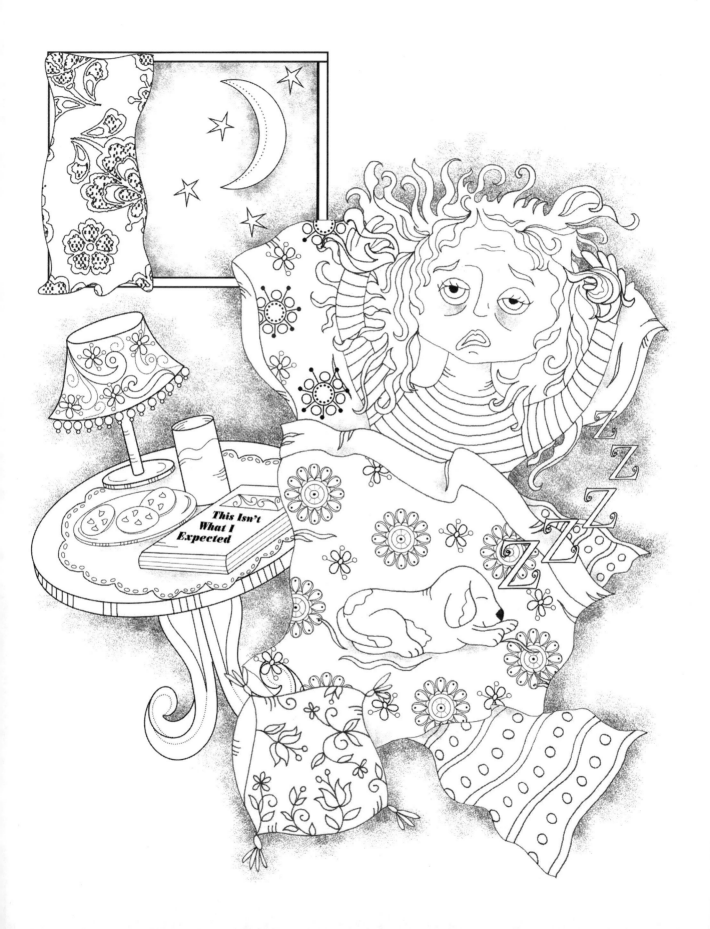

It's hard to put yourself on your list of things to take care of right now.
But you must.
Practice self-care, rest, take a walk.
Have some tea. Eat whatever tastes good.
Taking care of yourself is not a luxury.
It is essential.

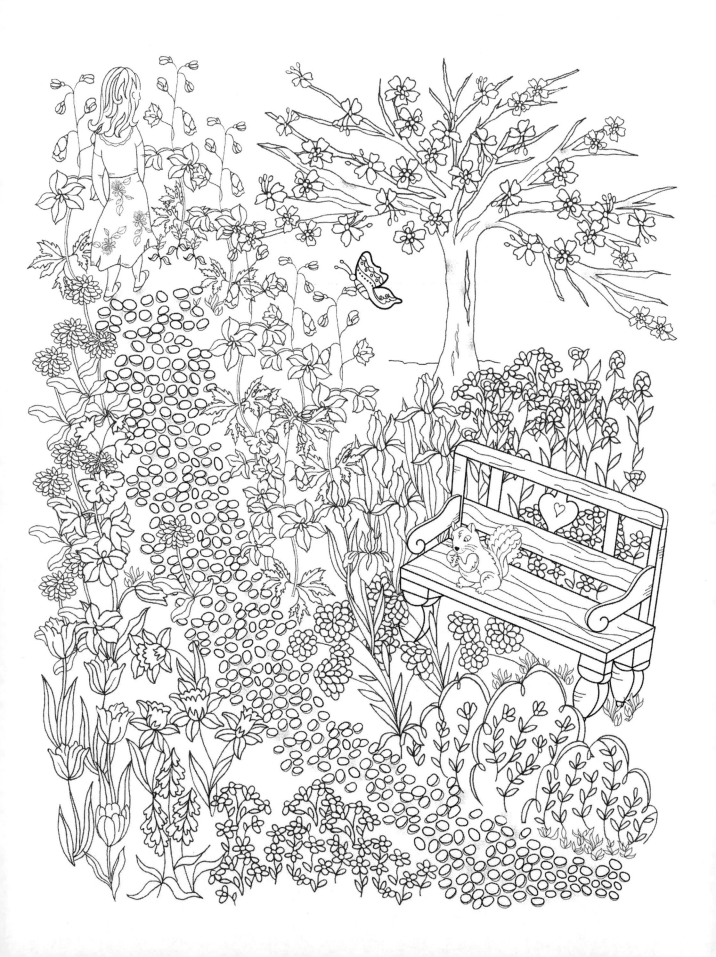

"I hope this goes away by itself. I don't want anyone to know."

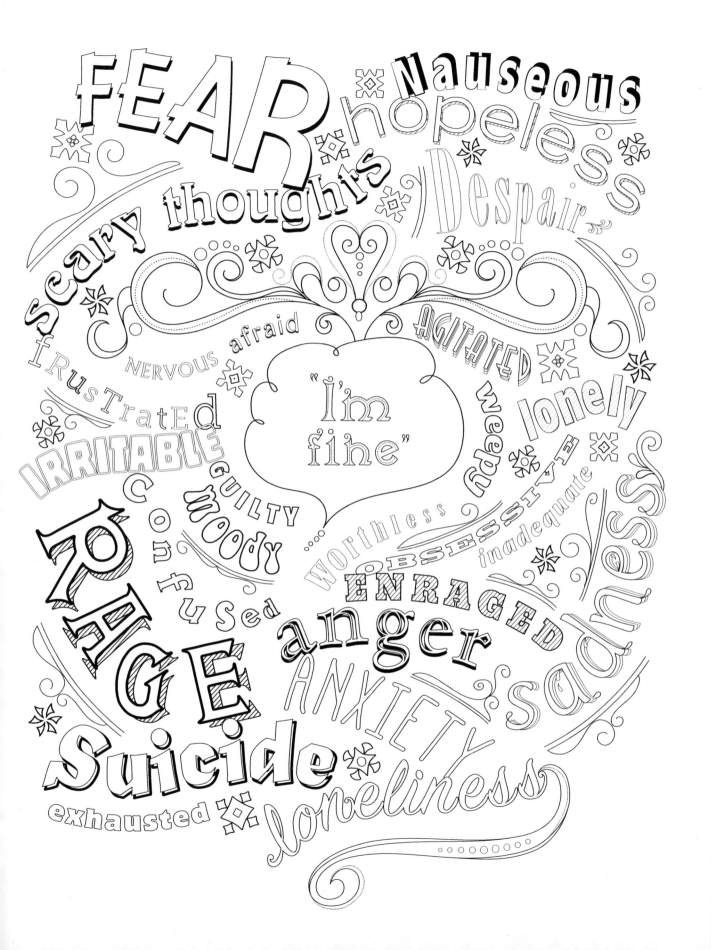

Asking for help is not a weakness.
Women who have been strong for too long get tired and depleted.
Asking for help is one of the best ways to replenish.
Reach out.

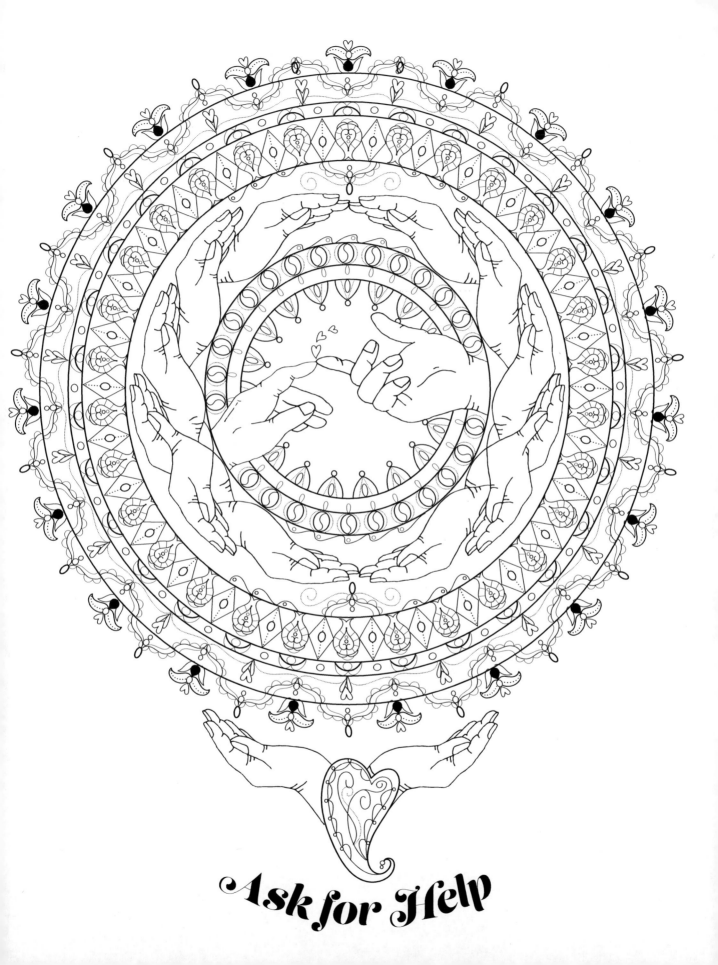

Ask for Help

"I feel nervous and totally overwhelmed."

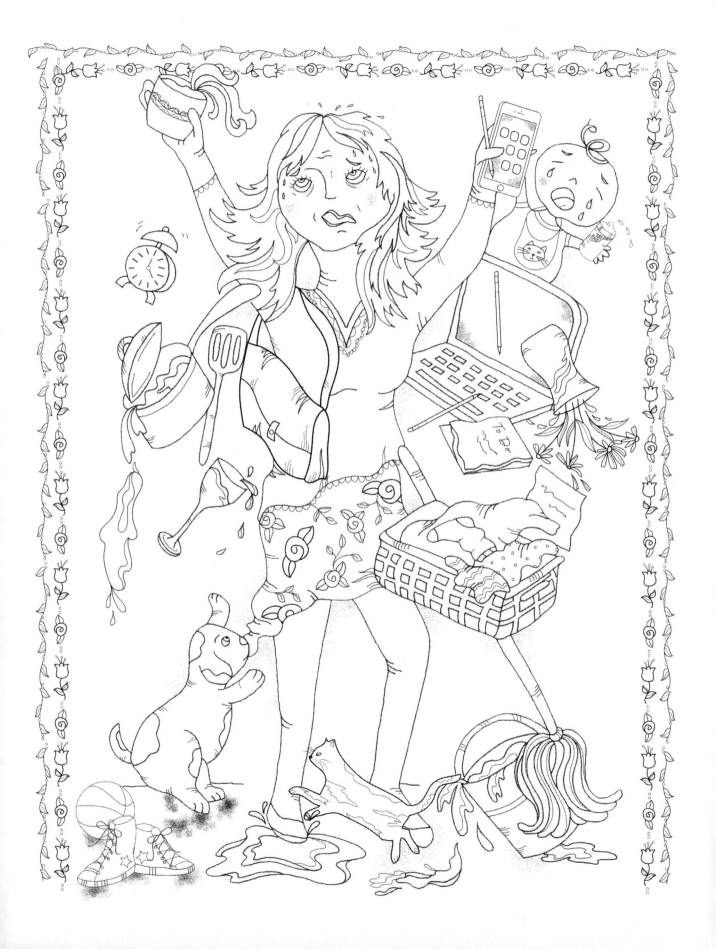

There is so much going on right now.
Avoid alcohol, caffeine, the Internet, and anthing that makes you feel bad.
Create a quiet space for yourself.
Make it your sanctuary.
Find 3 minutes. Breathe in and out slowly.
Really do it.

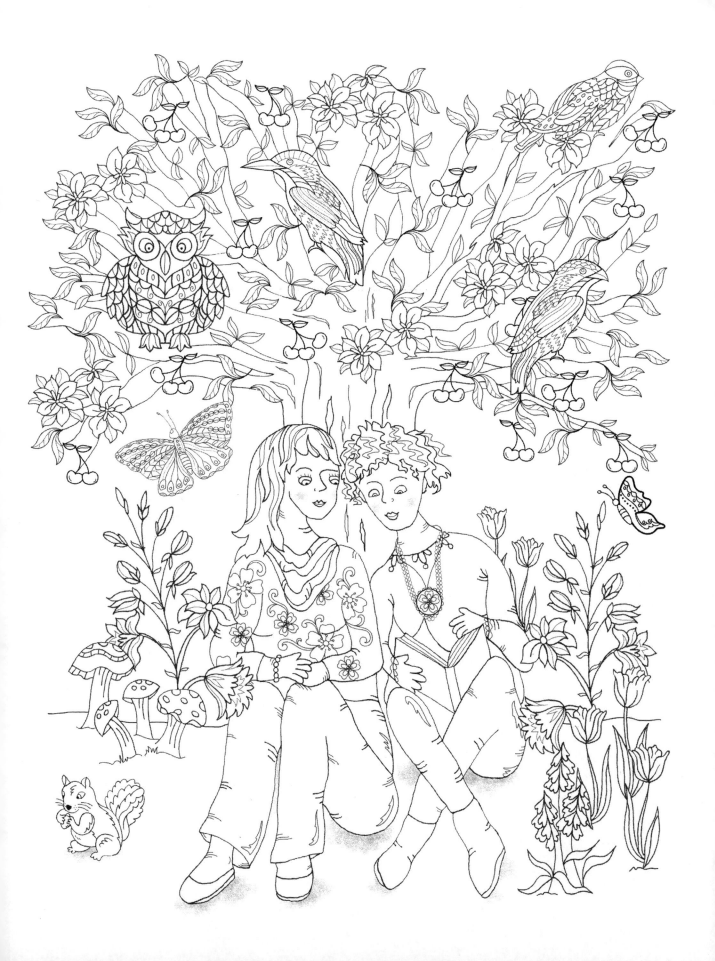

"My thoughts are racing. I cannot think. I just want to hide."

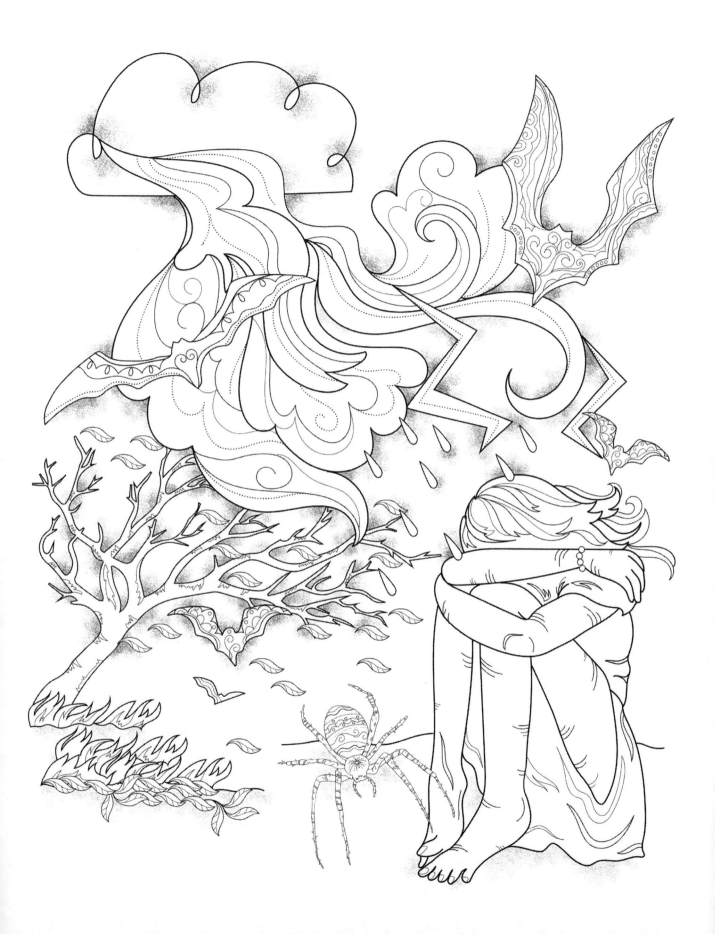

Sometimes it can feel so bad you don't know what to do.
Always let someone know how you feel.
Ground yourself with things that feel familiar and cozy.
Hugs are good. Keep your brain busy.
Count. Sing. Dance. Do a puzzle or numbers game.
Listen to music. Take a walk in the sunshine. Breathe. Play. Watch TV.
Sensory stimulations and distractions help the brain by concentrating on something else besides your worrisome thoughts.

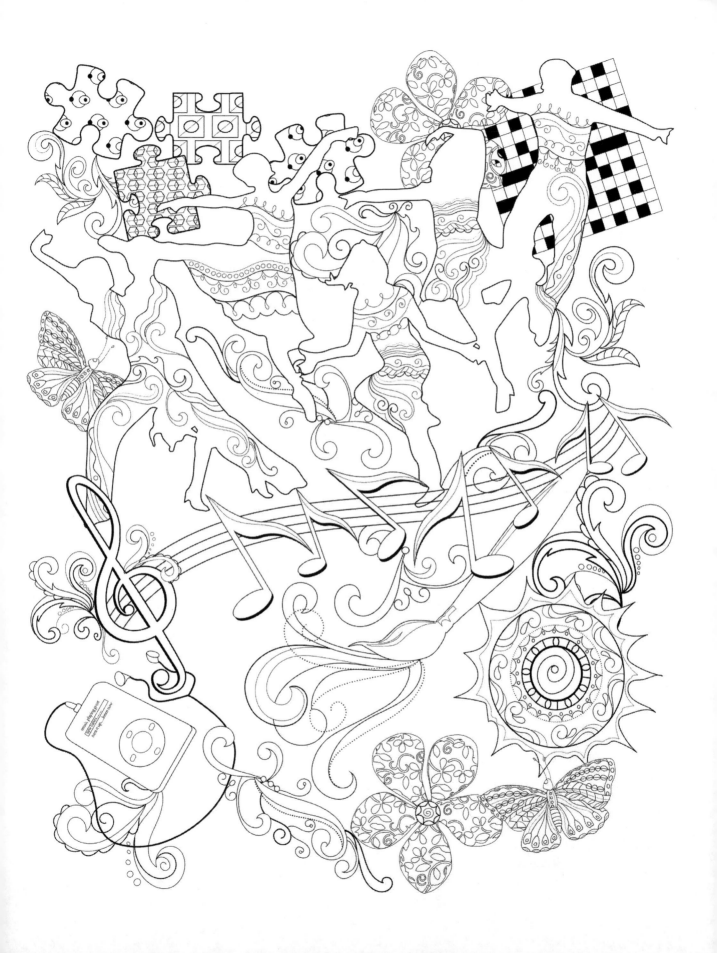

"I feel disconnected and detached."

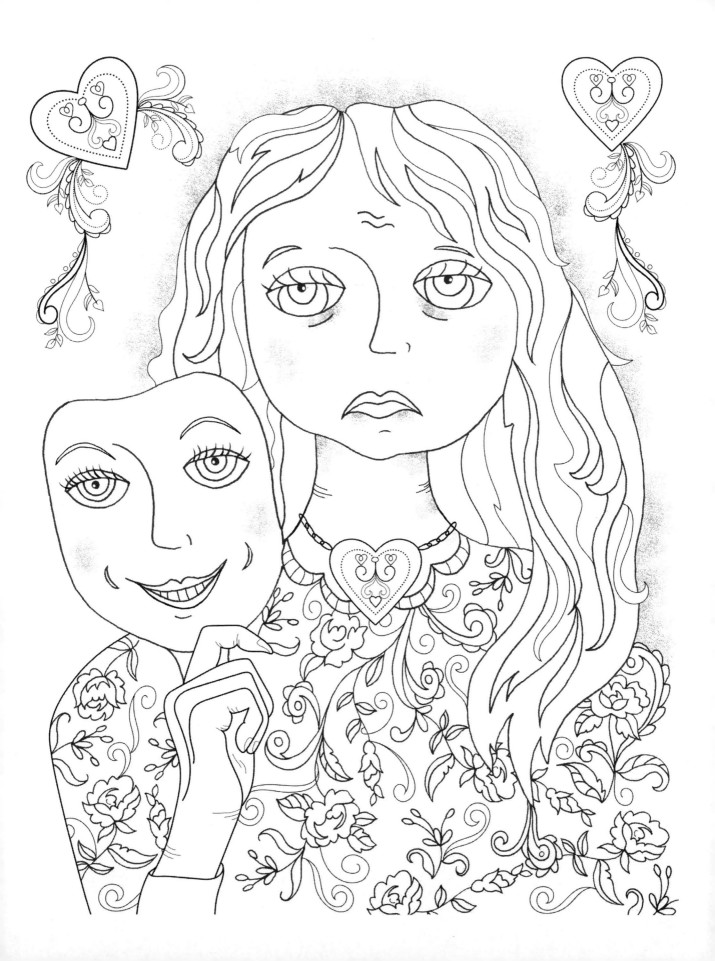

Whatever you feel right now is okay.
Nothing bad is happening.
Remind yourself you will not always feel this way.
Tell someone.

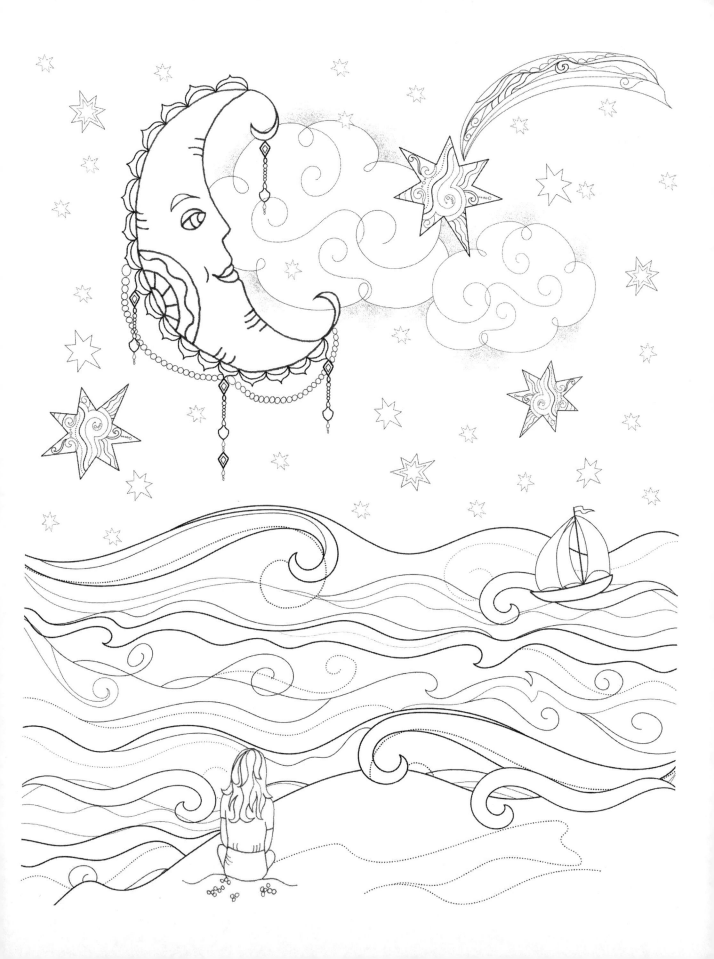

"I am so irritable. I hate everyone and everything."

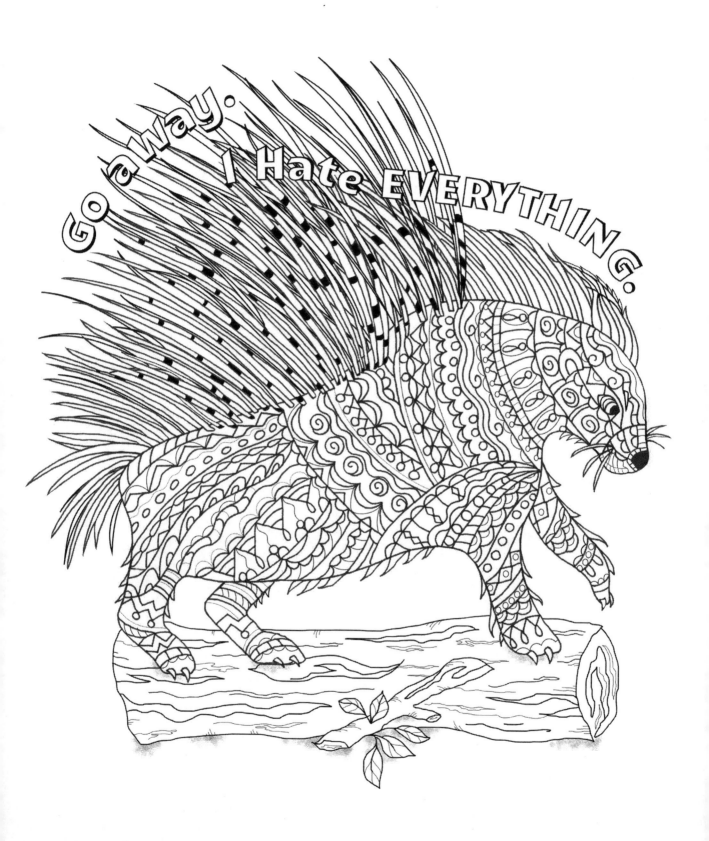

You are doing the best you can.
It's enough right now.
You are hanging in with your distress.
You are trying to believe in yourself.
Reward yourself for small achievements.

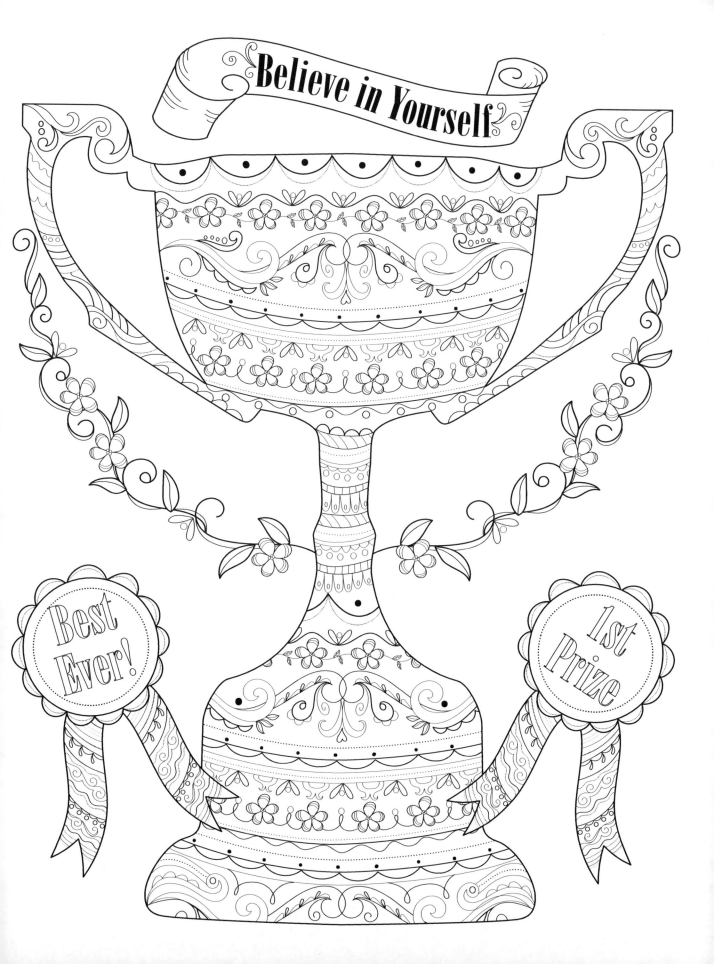

"Everything feels so hard. I feel unworthy, Inadequate and unfit to be a mother."

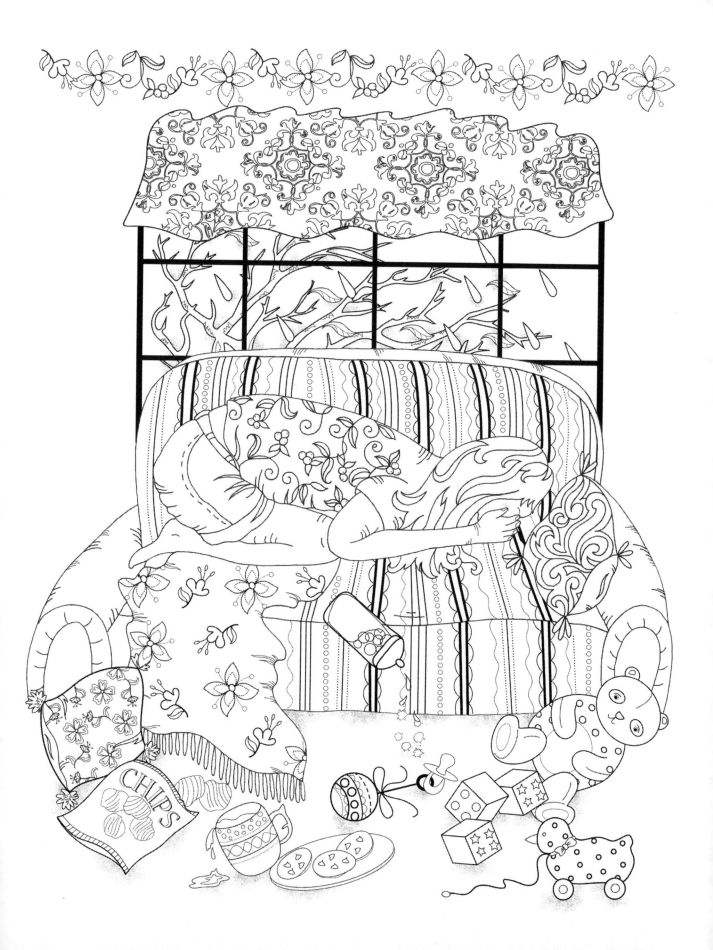

It's hard to be a mother sometimes.
Try to let go of wanting to do things perfectly.
Give yourself permission to expect less.
Good mothers have bad days.
Being a good-enough mother is good-enough.

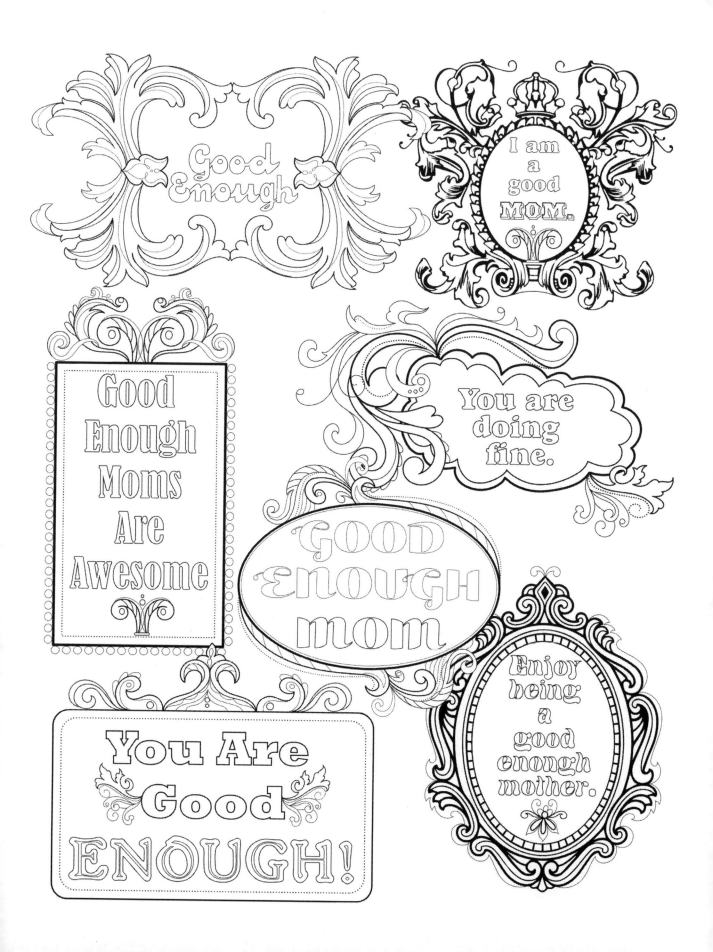

"I'm afraid to be alone but I don't feel like being with friends and family."

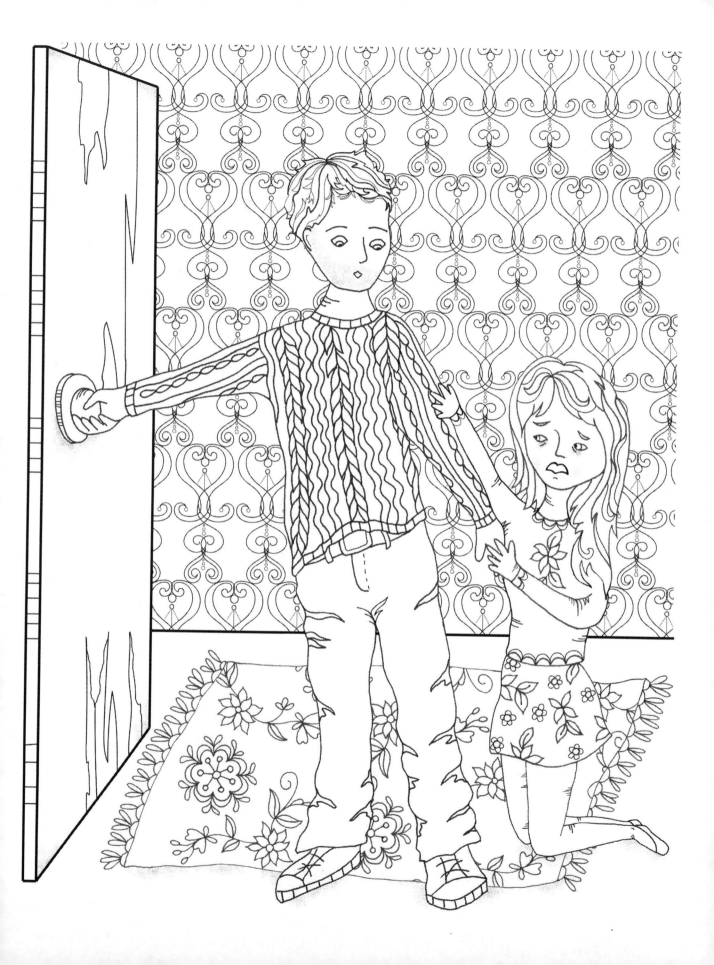

Surround yourself with people, places and things, which make you feel safe and loved.

Do not overwhelm yourself.

Take it slow when making plans.

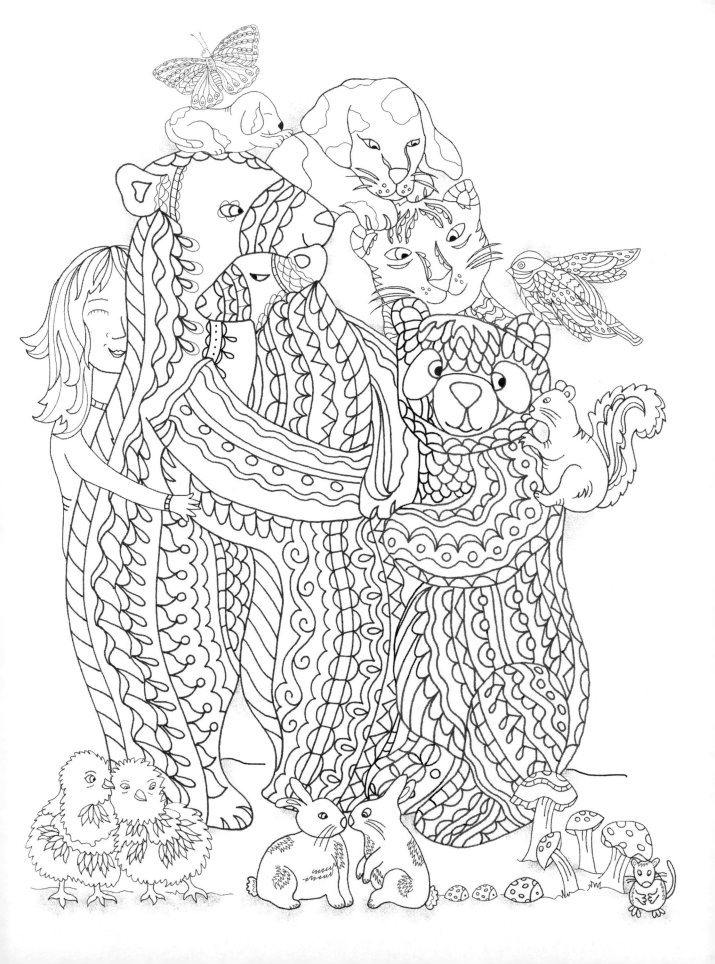

"I am constantly worried.
I keep asking the same questions over and over.
Now I am worried about my worrying."

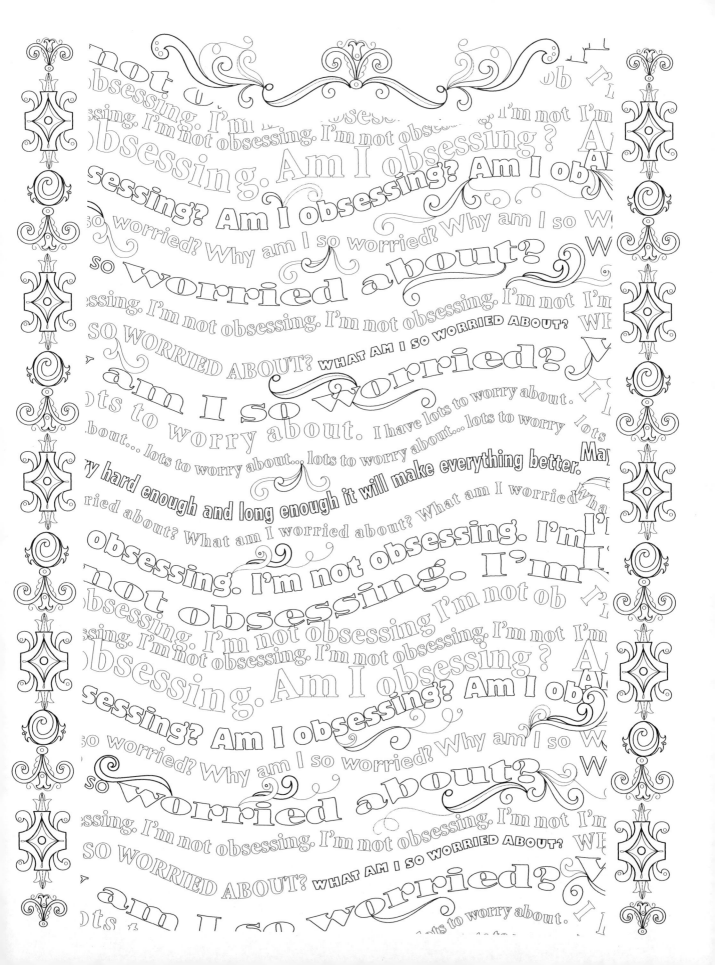

Most fears are based on perceived, rather than real threats.
There are lots of unknowns and living with uncertainty is hard.
You can learn to tolerate some anxiety without feeling out of control.
Smile more. Laugh loud.
Accept that anxiety is present.

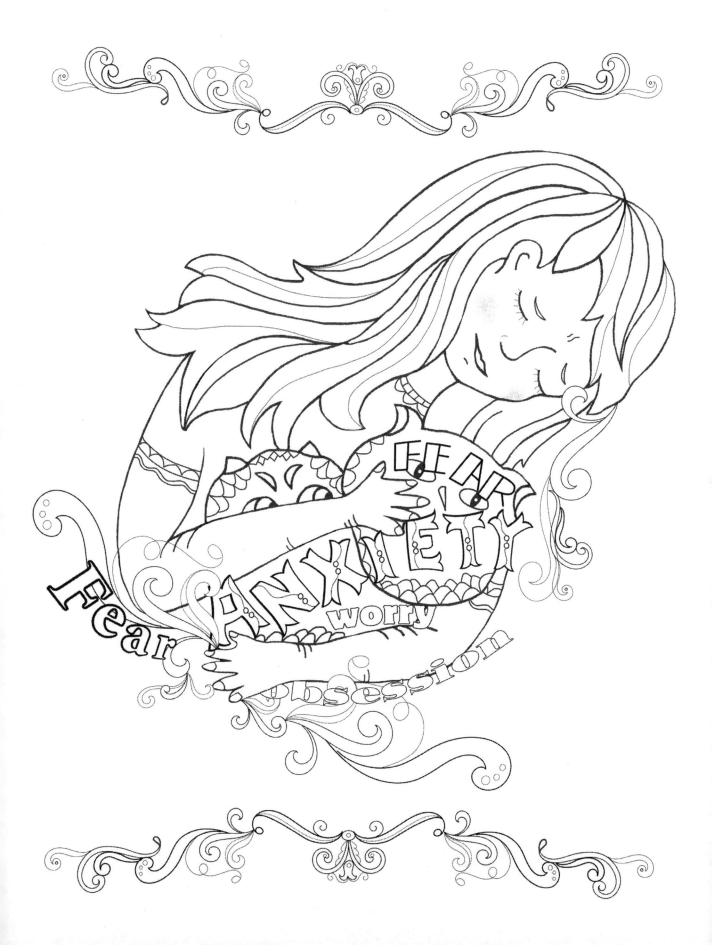

"I blame myself for everything. I can't do anything right."

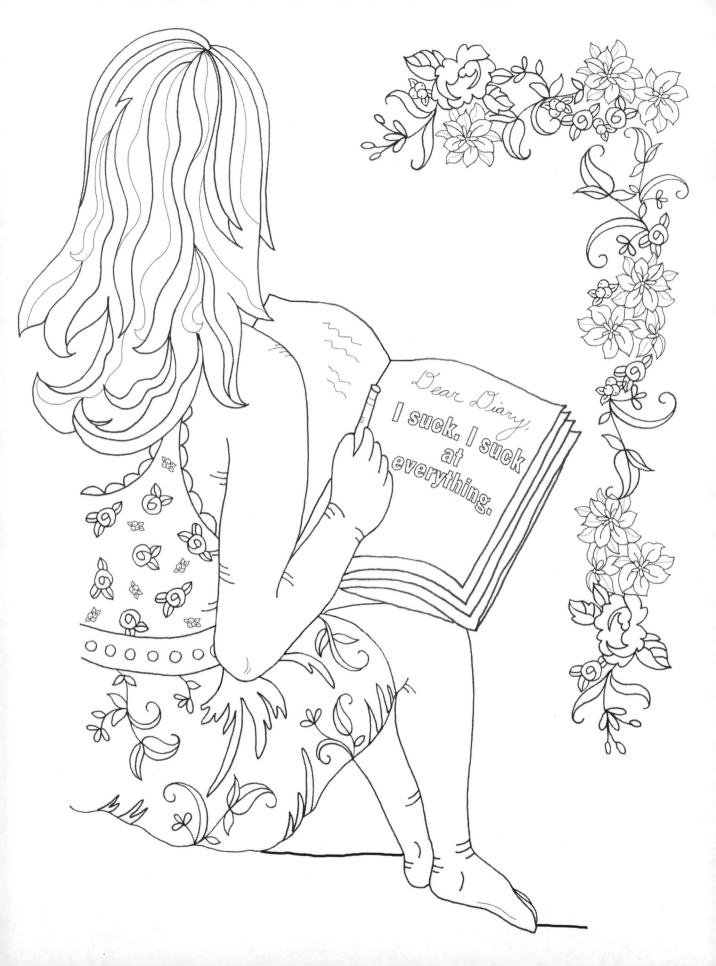

Guilt is common during this time.
Remind yourself that you are a good mother.
Good mothers make mistakes.
Try to find things you feel good about.

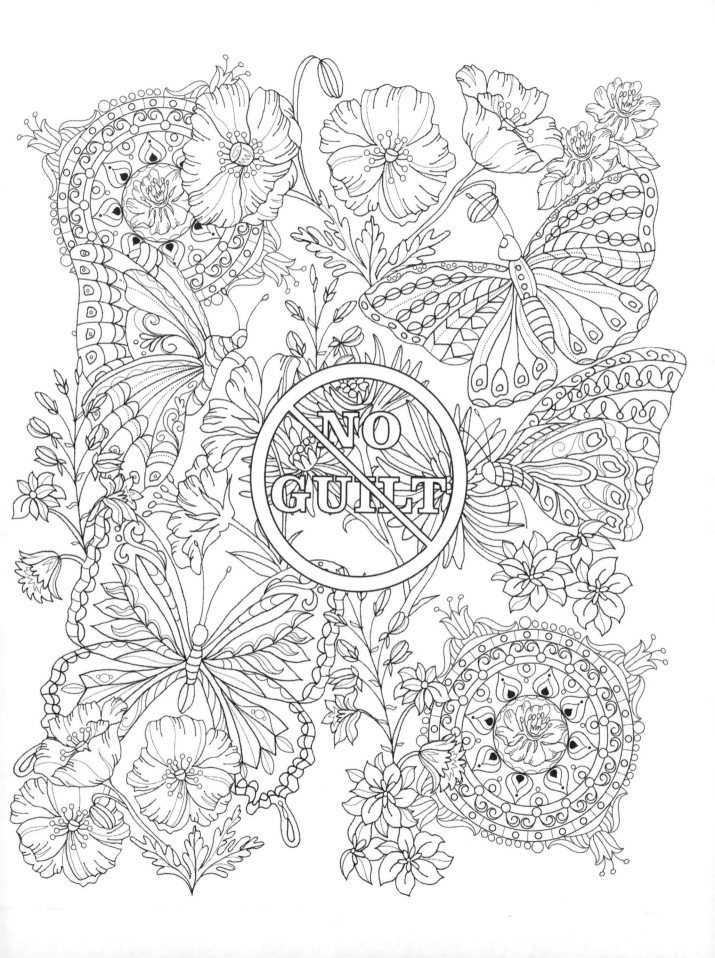

"My world feels unpredictable and out of control".

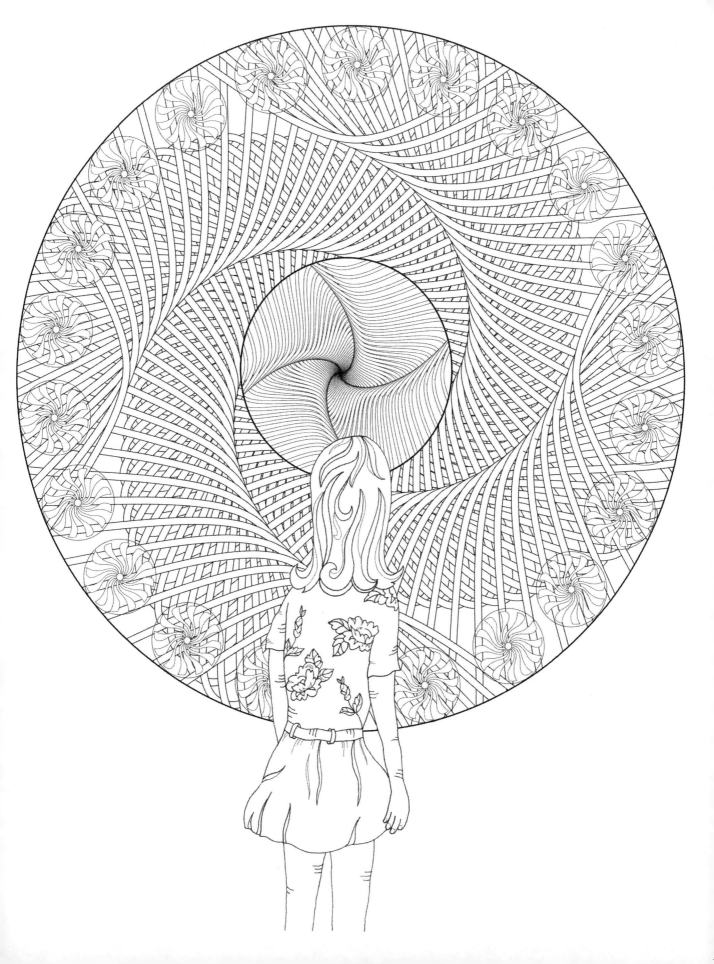

If you are worried about the way you are feeling or thinking, find a professional who can help you.
Symptoms of depression and anxiety are treatable.
One day soon, you will feel better.
You will feel like yourself again.

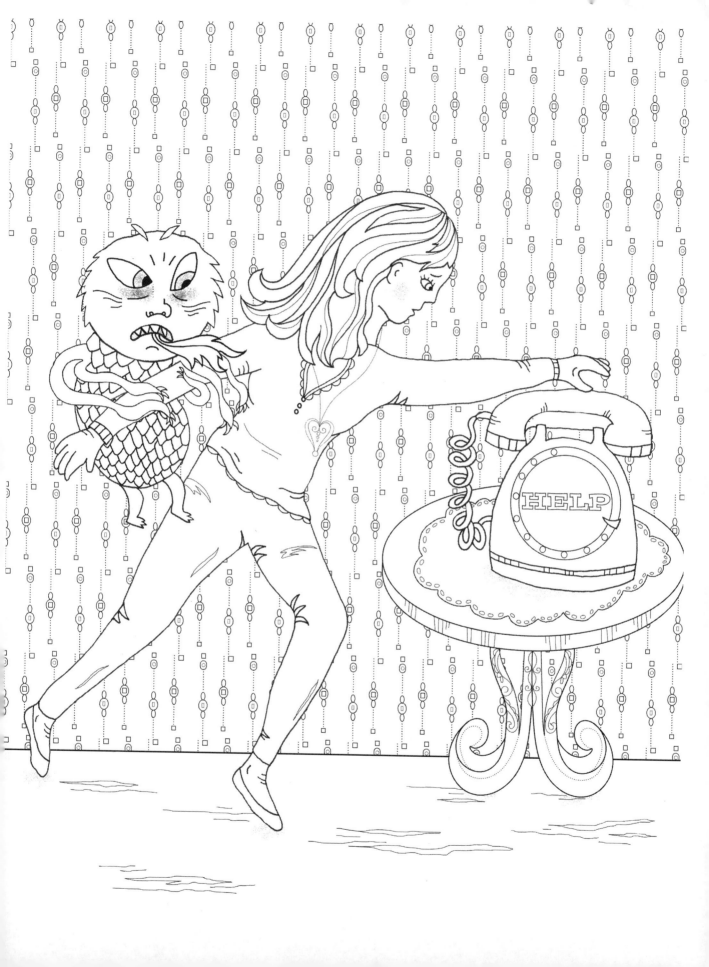

"I cannot find pleasure in anything. I feel empty inside. I'm afraid I will always feel this way. I've made a terrible mistake."

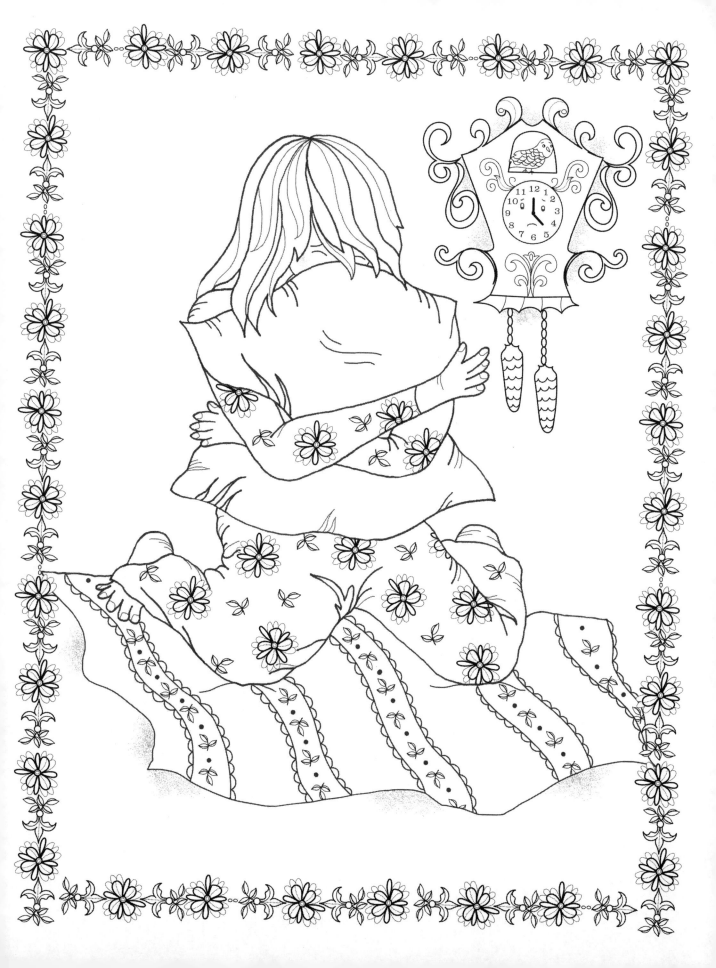

These feelings are symptoms.
You will not always feel this way.
You are okay.
Things will get better.

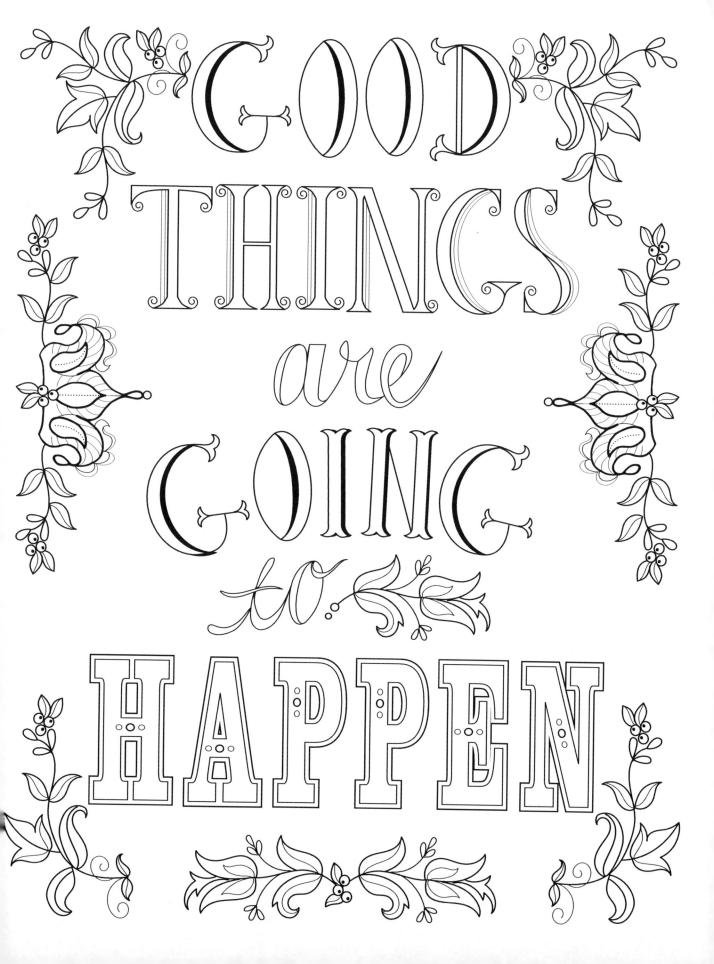

You are stronger than you know.

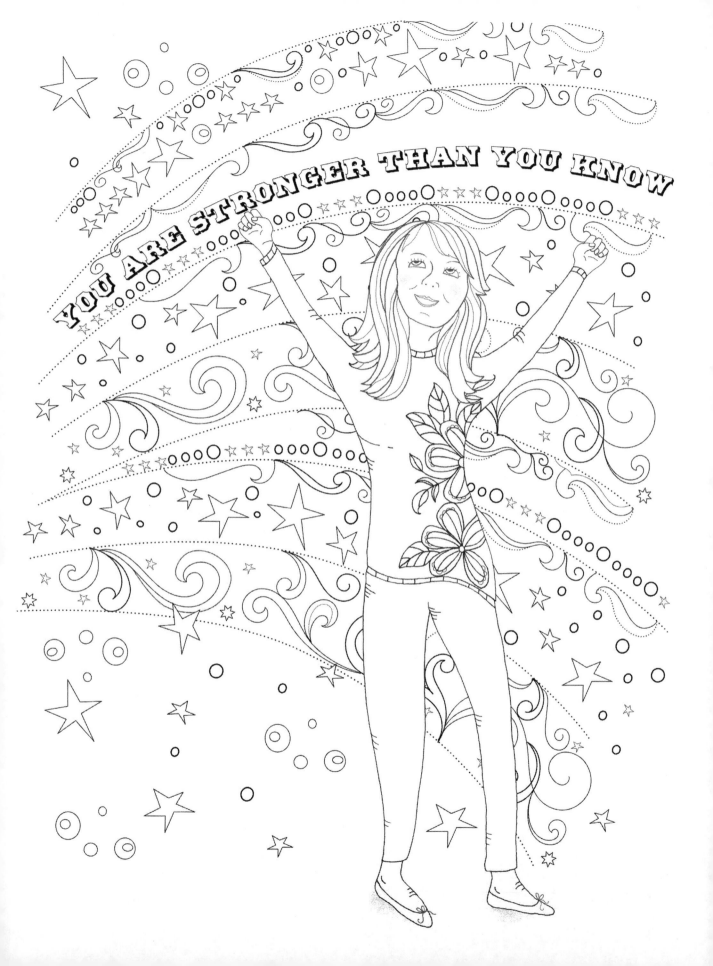

If you are worried about the way you are feeling or thinking, please find a professional who can help you feel better. If you can't find a speciali in your area, please visit THE POSTPARTUM STRESS CENTER *postpartumstress.com* or POSTPARTUM SUPPORT INTERNATIONAL *postpartum.ne* for referrals to experts in your area.

Made in the USA
Lexington, KY
29 June 2018